PMS

A Nutritional Approach

by Louise Tenney

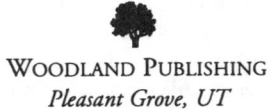

WOODLAND PUBLISHING
Pleasant Grove, UT

Contents

PMS: A Brief History

PMS is a phenomenon experienced by a great number of women. Its letters stand for Premenstrual Syndrome, a term which refers to a collection of symptoms which occur for these women prior to the onset of their menstrual period. It is also known as Premenstrual Tension. Over 150 ailments have been linked to PMS and more are emerging all the time. While science had a tendency to initially take PMS with a grain of salt, it is now accepted as a legitimate condition which can be responsible for a whole host of undesirable symptoms.

If severe enough, PMS can be very serious—not only for its victims, but for their families and friends as well. It quite obvious that PMS has most certainly reached the forefront of awareness when it can be legally used as a courtroom defense for assault and battery. Clearly, within the last 15 years, PMS has been officially recognized as a legitimate disorder that can have significant physical and mental effects on certain women.

PMS can affect any woman who has menstrual cycles and usually occurs one to two weeks prior to menstruation. It generally targets women between that ages of 24 and 40. It has been described as "a disorder that encompasses emotional, behavioral and physical symptoms." PMS has not just suddenly popped up over the last few years. It has been afflicting the female gender since the beginning of time, however, it remained unrecognized and unnamed for generations.

Women who suffered from PMS in the past were frequently labeled neurotic or even mentally ill, especially in extreme cases of PMS. Typically after hearing that their symptoms were "all in their heads," aspirin or tranquilizers would be prescribed to placate them. The very complex role that hormonal fluctuations exert on every system of the body was not understood by these physicians, many of whom even doubted the real existed of menstrual cramps.

The syndrome was first mentioned in professional journals during the 1930s, however it was not until the last two decades that PMS emerged into public discussions or medical diagnosis. It was not until two women in England were accused of murder and used PMS as a contributing factor that the syndrome began to receive the attention it merited. Over two million women in the United States suffer from PMS.

Today, public awareness has generated a great deal of publicity enabling women to openly seek and receive the help they need. A great wealth of information is available on PMS. Unfortunately, using natural therapies to manage the problem is rarely explored. While the artificial manipulation of hormones may be necessary in some cases of PMS, using nutritional and herbal treatments can affect dramatic changes for the better and in some cases, relieve the syndrome altogether.

Causes of PMS

PMS is considered a physiological condition which an occur from a hormonal imbalance or an sensitivity to certain hormone levels. High levels of estrogen which occur prior to the onset of menstruation can act as a stimulant to the central nervous system producing a variety of symptoms. Progesterone can help to balance the effects of estrogen, however, in some cases, progesterone levels decrease and hormonal levels become disrupted.

Other possible causes or contributing factors of PMS include: food allergies, low blood sugar levels, edema, yeast infections, lead poisoning, physical and mental stress, constipation and nutritional deficiencies. There is also some evidence to suggest that thyroid dysfunction can also cause PMS.

Dr. Guy E. Abraham, MD, a former professor of Obstetrics, Gynecology and Endocrinology at UCLA has done extensive research on PMS. He strongly believes that PMS is an illness caused by a hormonal imbalance, low blood sugar levels, edema, physical and mental stress and nutritional deficiencies.

Symptoms of PMS

PMS symptoms generally strike women between the ages of 25 and 40, although 40% of females between the ages of 14 and 50 can be prone to it. This endocrine disorder has appropriately been dubbed, "The Monthly Curse.î Over 150 different ailments have been attributed to PMS. The most common ones include abdominal bloating, water retention, breast swelling and tenderness, and mood changes such as irritability, depression and heightened anxiety. PMS is capable of causing mild to severe personality changes and dramatic mood swings. Symptoms of PMS occur cyclically and usually peak the week prior to menstruation. For many women, symptoms are the most severe two to five days prior to their periods and subside as the period progresses. PMS can occur up to two weeks before menstruation and forms of PMS can develop on the last day of the menstrual cycle in some women. Some women only experience PMS in mild enough forms that it poses no real problem. For others, the syndrome is severe enough to significantly compromise the quality of life.

PHYSICAL SYMPTOMS ASSOCIATED WITH PMS

Menstrual cramps
Abdominal Bloating
Water Retention
Skin Eruptions
Headaches
Backache
Breast Enlargement
Breast Tenderness
Increased Appetite
Food Cravings
Fatigue
Insomnia
Candida

Joint Pain
Weight Gain
Constipation or Diarrhea
Heart Palpitations
Low Blood Sugar
Rhinitis
Dizziness
Heavy Menstrual Flow
Allergies
Fainting
Asthma
Eye Infections (Conjunctivitis)

PSYCHOLOGICAL SYMPTOMS ASSOCIATED WITH PMS

Depression
Lethargy
Irritability
Agitation
Sleep Disturbances
Nervousness
Short Temper/Violent Outbursts
Withdrawal of Affection

Nervous Tension
Forgetfulness
Disorientation
Crying Spells
Erratic Behavior
Anxiety
A Desire to Run Away
Suicidal Thoughts

Symptoms of PMS can be divided into distinct categories. They are;

A) *Behavioral:* These symptoms deal with psychological changes and can involve mild to severe personality changes which are characterized by one or several of the behaviors listed above.

B) *Neurological:* Headaches, including migraines are the most prevalent neurological symptoms of PMS, however, dizziness can also occur.

C) *Respiratory:* PMS can cause an increased incidence of colds or promote the onset of allergic reactions such as rhinitis and in some cases asthma.

D) *Gastrointestinal:* PMS is not commonly associated with a number of gastrointestinal disorders, however, it can be a significant factor in abdominal bloating, diarrhea, constipation, appetite fluctuations and even colitis.

E) *Other:* Edema, temporary weight gain, heart fluttering, acne, breast tissue enlargement, skin bruising and eye infections and irritations can also be caused by PMS.

Do You Have PMS?

Sometimes it can be difficult to assess if you have a true case of PMS. Dr. Robert W. Downs, DC, has offered these tips and advice for women who want to know if their cycle is responsible for the way they feel. "I suggest that women chart their symptoms very carefully for at least two months. Use a calendar and mark when each symptom begins and ends. Weigh each morning to see if fluid retention occurs. Ask a family member to observe and record mood changes." After recording the above information for several months, answer the following questions:

A) *Are your symptoms occurring between ovulation and menstruation?*
B) *Do the symptoms start after a significant hormonal change such as puberty, pregnancy, starting or stopping birth control pills, or missed periods or tubal ligation?*
C) *Do the symptoms become worse after a second hormonal change?*
D) *Do family and friends notice a change in your behavior before menstruation?*

If you have answered yes to all or all but one of these questions, you probably suffer from PMS.

Hormonal Culprits of PMS

High levels of estrogen and lower levels of progesterone have been linked to PMS. Estrogen is naturally produced in the ovaries along with progesterone. While estrogen can act as a nervous system stimulant, progesterone works as a depressant. For this reason, the right levels of each of these hormones creates a balance. If levels of progesterone become too low, the hormonal scales will tip in favor of estrogen. It is this specific imbalance which appears to precipitate PMS.

Some doctors will approach PMS by prescribing synthetic progesterone which is taken during that last part of the menstrual cycle. Oral contraceptives, anti-prostaglandins and diuretics are also routinely used to treat PMS. The use of synthetic hormonal therapy can provide temporary relief, however the side effects of such drugs are substantial. Nutritional and herbal treatments can be very effective and should be implemented before synthetic hormones are used. Some of the side effects of hormonal drugs include: chest pains, abnormal menstrual bleeding, vaginal and rectal swelling, and disruptions of weight. The increased risk of cancer has also been associated with the use of synthetic hormones.

Progesterone occurs in several plants such as wild yam and sarsaparilla in their natural steroid form. Natural progesterone is rarely used by doctors who prefer stronger, artificial pharmaceutical versions of the hormone. Interestingly, natural forms of progesterone are considered anti-carcinogenic substances, while synthetic forms have been linked to an increased cancer risk. One very important fact to remember is that the ratio of estrogen and progesterone is more critical than the actual levels of these two hormones in the body. Achieving a balance between estrogen and progesterone naturally will be discussed in more detail in a later section of this booklet.

THE ROLE OF BLOOD SUGAR LEVELS

PMS can create a form of temporary hypoglycemia or low blood sugar. For this reason, some women will experience dramatic cravings for sugar just prior to their periods. Food binging on carbohydrates and cravings for chocolate are typical. In addition, erratic behavior that can be triggered by low blood sugar compounds other PMS symptoms. This type of hypoglycemia is linked to shifts in the ratio between estrogen and progesterone.

When elevated levels of estrogen occur, more insulin is released into the bloodstream lowering blood sugar levels, therefore prompting the urge to eat. Unfortunately, eating sugar to relieve "sugar blues" only makes matters worse. Sugar raises blood sugar levels quickly which initiates more insulin and the cycle continues. In addition, if sugar is heavily consumed. It can leech calcium out of the bones and teeth. B-vitamins which are crucial in helping the body avoid mood swings and depression are destroyed by a high sugar intake. Increased irritability has been associated with sugar binging. Diet changes in combination with herbal and vitamin supplementation can help to prevent the strong sugar cravings so typical of PMS. In addition to hormonal imbalances, nutrient depletion can also contribute to erratic eating.

Dr. Richard Wurtman, a professor of neuroscience and specialist in brain chemistry in conjunction with his wife, Judith, compiled some fascinating data on women who suffer from PMS. We know that women who suffer from PMS typically crave carbohydrates or sugar. The Wurtmans discovered that a drop in serotonin levels in the brain can create a carbohydrate craving. Eating carbohydrates helps to bring up serotonin levels thus improving mood.

CHOCOLATE CRAVINGS AND PMS

The Wurtman Study also found that one of the common denominators in all cases of PMS was a magnesium deficiency. Chocolate contains magnesium; however, it is also high in caffeine and fat. Chocolate also contains phenylalanine, an amino acid which is needed for healthy brain activity. This amino acid has amphetamine-like properties which actually act as natural antidepressants. Women who suffer from severe cases of PMS can crave chocolate so intensely that they will ransack the house searching for even an old stale chocolate. A plunging mood can prompt this search for chocolate and is the body's way of trying to combat depression.

ESTROGEN AND DEPRESSION

High levels of estrogen can actually produce depression. Combined with the effects of low blood sugar, this depression can become quite serious. Some women who take birth control pills refer to them as "grouch pills" because they typically cause moodiness. It is vital to stress, at this point, that most of us believe that we are eating right and getting enough vitamins and minerals. The truth is that many of us suffer from a lack of certain nutrients that we desperately need to fight PMS.

Excess estrogen can create a shortage of tryptophan or vitamin B6 which are both needed to keep serotonin in the brain at optimal levels. It is not uncommon for women who take estrogen to relive the symptoms of menopause to battle periods of depression due to vitamin B6 depletion.

While science is beginning to understand PMS as a complex biological phenomenon, its intrinsic connection to nutrition has not been investigated by the medical community as a whole. PMS is a disorder caused by a biochemical imbalance. Frequently, a disruption in body chemistry can be successfully treated with certain vitamins like therapeutic doses of vitamin B6.

WATER RETENTION

A rise in estrogen can also promote fluid buildup in the tissues due to its ability to attract salt, which in turn, attracts water. PMS can cause swelling in the tissues of the stomach, breasts, legs and even the brain. Diuretics are routinely used to prevent water retention but can inadvertently cause more stress on the body. Diuretics can leech out vital minerals such as potassium and magnesium along with the excess water. A depletion of these minerals can promote cramping in the legs, feet, and hands. Some diuretics contain other undesirable substances like aspirin and/or ammonium chloride which can also upset the body's delicate chemistry even further. Natural diuretics, which are discussed in a later section of this book are much safer in that the work with the body rather than against it.

STRESS

Most of us will agree that we live with too much stress. Unfortunately, stress is here to stay, however our ability to manage stress can be enhanced. Stress, whether physical or mental increases our need for vitamins and minerals. Nutrients are more quickly depleted when the body experiences periods of stress. If these nutrients are not replenished regularly, the body is left without the benefit of these vital catalysts which help to maintain normal hormonal activity.

Stress can adversely affect the body is several ways. Stress taxes our immune system making us more susceptible to disease. It can cause emotional problems and most certainly aggravates PMS. We live is a hurry up and wait world and typically rush to get kids off to school, fight traffic, run to keep appointments, worry about family pressures, financial stressors etc. etc. Sadly, it is during periods of high stress that most of us fail to eat and sleep properly, placing even more stress on our physiology. We need to stop and pay attention to our nutrition. Becoming low in certain vitamins and minerals only serves to ad fuel to the PMS fire.

Nutritional Deficiencies and PMS

The main thrust of this booklet is to point out that nutritional deficiencies lie at the heart of PMS. RDA standards are not adequate levels to enable the body cope or correct physiological conditions such as PMS. In addition, many of us suffer from a lack of nutrients we assumed we were getting plenty of. Studies have shown that women with PMS tend to consume less B vitamins, half as much zinc and iron, one fourth a much manganese and more dairy products, salt, sugar, protein and animal fat than other women.

Most of us have experienced the gnawing and persistent hunger associated with PMS. Extreme hunger and food binging seems to occur when estrogen and progesterone levels are at their highest. It is common during these phases for women to consume more than double their regular calorie intake.

It has been proven that a diet which is deficient in calcium, magnesium and B6 can trigger PMS symptoms such as irritability, edema, etc. A diet rich in fresh fruits and vegetables, whole grains, beans, peas, lentils, nuts and seeds, broiled chicken, turkey or fish helps to control PMS. This regimen involves the kind of smart eating all of us should incorporate into our lives whether we suffer form PMS or not. It focuses on foods rich in vitamins, minerals, and complex carbohydrates.

FOODS TO EMPHASIZE FOR PMS

Because women who suffer from PMS typically crave carbohydrates, it is very important that instead of chips and cookies, foods that are slowly digested and low in fat should be eaten instead. When you crave a carb, reach for raw seeds or nuts, which act to supply the body with protein and help to stabilize blood sugar levels. Once this happens, the desire to binge will subside, helping to prevent the weight gain which can routinely occur when estrogen levels are high.

Foods to emphasize are: brown rice, lentils, potatoes, beans of all kinds, split peas, millet, whole grain breads, cereals and pasta, fresh/raw vegetables and fruits, lean, white meats, high fiber foods, blackstrap molasses, sesame seeds, sunflower seeds, and raw almonds.

Foods and substances to avoid include: white sugar, caffeine, chocolate, alcohol, salty foods, fatty foods, high fat dairy products, red meats, hydrogenated oils, saturated fats, fatty/sugary snacks (chips, cookies, pastries), nicotine/tobacco, diuretics, salt, chlorinated water, and birth control pills.

Did you know that salt can cause irritability, breast tenderness and water retention. When salt is combined with sugar, the problem is compounded even more causing an increase in pain and swelling. Some studies have found that caffeine can also contribute to the formation of breast enlargement and even breast tumors. It also contributes to calcium loss. Nicotine destroys nutrients in the body and should be avoided like the plague. It is a clearly a drug and causes addiction leading to a whole host of life threatening diseases, not to mention constant nutrient depletion. Alcohol poisons the liver and interferes with the action of vitamins and minerals. It also leeches calcium from the body. White sugar robs the body of magnesium and B vitamins and can cause abrupt fluctuations in blood sugar levels which causes irritability and mood changes. While dairy products may seem desirable for their calcium content, they contain high amount of calcium without the presence of magnesium. This can actually contribute to the excretion of magnesium from the body, causing anxiety and nervousness. Chlorinated water seems harmless enough; however, it can destroy the action of vitamin E which is so crucial to normalizing hormonal levels. Fatty foods also interfere with magnesium absorption and can trigger uterine cramping.

RED MEAT: ITS HIDDEN DANGERS

Red meats should be eaten very sparingly or altogether avoided. Cattle are routinely fed antibiotics and sex-growth hormones which can be passed on to humans. It is thought that the high prevalence of hormonal imbalances in humans may be triggered by the ingestion of meat and milk which contain these hormones. Obesity, diabetes, kidney disease, hypoglycemia, and masculinization of females and the feminization of males, and cancer may be related to the ingestion of these animal hormones.

Some doctors strongly suspect that a link exists between the hormones found in meat and milk and increased breast and uterine soreness experienced by so many women today. Likewise, it is thought that obesity may be promoted by the hormones used to fatten cattle. In addition, cattle routinely eat grain/grasses exposed to high levels of pesticides, herbicides and other toxins.

The medical establishment has finally accepted that red meat can contribute to heart disease and certain types of cancer due to its high saturated fat content. It has not yet acknowledged these other potentially life threatening drawbacks of red meat. Eating an excess of red meant can profoundly disturb hormonal function, and balance, contributing to severe PMS symptoms. Interestingly, vegetarian women, who get adequate B vitamins have lower blood levels of estradiol, a form of estrogen which can actually cause tumors and other undesirable side effects.

Minerals for PMS

Calcium: Blood calcium levels can drop ten days prior to menstruation. This occurs when the ovaries are not producing large amounts of estrogen or progesterone and can continue even after the menstrual period has ceased. This steady decline in calcium levels can cause tension, headaches, nervousness, cramping, insomnia and depression. The addition of magnesium and vitamin D to calcium enhance its absorption. Several herbs such as oat straw, horsetail, comfrey, and lobelia are naturally high in calcium. In addition these herbs contain silicon, which also facilitates better calcium absorption. Remember, you can take all the calcium supplements in the store, but if you are not absorbing that calcium, it is excreted in the body's waste and serves no beneficial purpose.

Magnesium: Magnesium also helps to relieve cramps, calms the nervous system and is a blood clotting agent. It also helps to prevent spasms in the uterine walls and leg muscles. In addition, magnesium increases the absorption of B-complex vitamins which helps to rid the body of excess estrogen, thereby preventing irritability and depression.

Zinc: Zinc helps to stabilize blood sugar levels which contribute to carbohydrate cravings. It also helps to regulate and release prostaglandin's which are substances which help to control uterine cramping. Zinc also helps to prevent hormonal imbalance.

Iron: Many women who have a heavy menstrual flow can become anemic. Taking a good, readily absorbable iron supplement is recommended for preventing anemia, and combating fatigue, weakness and depression which originates form a low red blood cell count. Taking vitamin C with iron is desirable as it helps the body assimilate iron.

Chromium Chromium contributes to blood sugar stabilization, much like zinc and works to keep blood sugar levels stable by promoting normal insulin activity.

Iodine: Iodine contributes to thyroid health and is closely involved in the production of thyroxin which also works to balance hormones. Thyroxin helps to keep estrogen levels from climbing too high and also assists the body in regulating the menstrual cycle and avoiding excess water retention.

Selenium: Selenium is very good for treating menstrual cramps and breast tenderness. It also boosts the action of the immune system.

Potassium: Potassium is an electrolyte which works to regulate water balance in the tissues. Eating too much salt or sodium can result in a potassium deficiency and promote edema or water weight gain. The use of diuretics can also flush potassium stores from the body.

Vitamins for PMS

Vitamin A: Vitamin A helps to provide healthy mucous membranes such as those that line the reproductive organs. Vitamin A is also necessary for proper endocrine function and also works to help prevent or treat acne that can result from hormonal fluctuations. Taking the vitamin during the second half of the menstrual cycle seems more effective.

Vitamin C: This vitamin promotes the healing of cells and tissue. It is also good for alleviating stress due to its ability to fortify the adrenal glands. The C-Complex should include bioflavonoids which work to strengthen capillary walls which helps to prevent hemorrhaging. Vitamin C is also a safe and natural diuretic for water retention typically seen with PMS. It also contributes to the regulation of the menstrual flow and can help to relieve menstrual pain. Because this vitamin is not stored in the body, it must be constantly replenished through diet or supplementation. In addition, environmental toxins, smog, infections, etc. also deplete vitamin C.

Vitamin E: Vitamin E is absolutely essential to maintain the health of the reproductive system. It works to alleviate breast tenderness, fibrocystic breast disease, reduced fluid retention and eases cramping. Vitamin E is also very important for the healthy production and proper metabolism of sex hormones like estrogen and progesterone. It has also reduced nervous tension, headaches, fatigue, depression and insomnia.

Vitamin D: Vitamin D helps the body properly absorb calcium which is essential to calm the nerves, and to prevent insomnia and muscle cramping.

B-Complex: The B vitamins play a crucial role in preventing PMS and its related symptoms. It was in the early 1940s that the relationship between vitamin B complex depletion and menstrual cramps, PMS and fibrocystic disease was made. Clinical studies have shown that the amount of estrogen metabolized by the liver can be controlled with a sufficient intake of B vitamins. B-Complex is crucial for anyone who suffers from PMS. It helps prevent excess estrogen and also contributes to the proper metabolism of estrogen. If the diet is deficient in B vitamins, estrogen can accumulate in the breast and uterine tissue, increasing the risk of cancer. B vitamins also help to prevent depression, fatigue, sugar cravings, weight gain and bloating. Lack of Vitamin B2 combined with stress can result in depression, hysteria, trembling and extreme fatigue.

The B vitamins that are specifically linked to estrogen and its conversion are: choline, inositol, lecithin, B6, and B12. The first three are particularly useful in preventing fatty deposits in the liver. This is important because a liver that has been infiltrated with these deposits cannot metabolize estrogen properly. Inositol helps to combat anxiety and depression. It is B6, however, that is the primary alleviator of PMS distress. Dr. Guy Abraham, M.D., found in working with patients at UCLA that the use of B6 initiated relief for over 50 women suffering from PMS. Prior to taking the vitamin, these women experienced anxiety, nervousness, insomnia, breast tenderness, menstrual cramps and acne. Therapeutic doses of vitamin B6 ranging from 200 to 800 mgs. daily resulted in a marked decrease of these symptoms, including the disappearance of breast lumps. While B6 was used in higher amounts, it is important to know that all of the B vitamins should be taken in balanced dosages to insure the best response. In some cases, the increased dosage of a single nutrient is necessary to induce a specific physiological response.

Folic Acid: Folic acid is actually another very essential B vitamin which works to fortify the reproductive organs and helps prevent depression related to nutrient deficiencies.

Pantothenic Acid: This B vitamin should be added for its ability to support the adrenal glands which help in coping with stress.

Herbs for PMS

Botanical therapies have been considered natural food treatments which do not have the deleterious side effects of synthetic drugs. Herbs are particularly valuable because they not only have the ability to remedy disease, they work to rebuild body tissues and organs as well. When it comes to PMS, herbal treatments are particularly desirable because they can stimulate and nourish the specific organs which supply estrogen and progesterone. The following herbs are excellent for the treatment and the prevention of PMS symptoms and other related female disorders:

Black Cohosh: This herb contains natural hormonal components with steroidal components which help with menstrual cramping and delayed flow. Black Cohosh also provides the body with calcium and magnesium, considered nervine minerals which calm the nervous system.

Blessed Thistle: This botanical has traditionally been used to treat cramping and assist in achieving hormonal balance.

Cascara Sagrada: A gentle and effective natural laxative which helps to promote regularity and improve colon muscle tone.

Cramp Bark: This herb is recognized as a uterine sedative and antispasmodic, therefore it is highly recommended for menstrual cramping. Of all the herbs, cramp bark is the best natural uterine relaxant.

Dong Quai: Dong Quai has been used for generations as a botanical treatment for any female complaint. In China, the herb constitutes the base of any herbal combination or formula used to treat female disorders. It can help to relieve vaginal dryness, pain, bloating and depression. Dong Quai also provides nourishment for the blood and female glands and is referred to as "the queen of all female herbs."

Evening Primrose Oil: This herbal oil is derived from the willow female and can help with breast tenderness, mood changes, anxiety, irritability, headaches and fluid retention, all typical symptoms of PMS. It is rich in potassium and GLA (gamma-linolenic acid). This substance is vital for glandular health due to its ability to stimulate the body to create hormone-like compounds necessary for the proper functioning of specific organs. Prostaglandins also known as "miracle molecules" are found in Evening Primrose Oil and help alleviate menstrual cramping, fight depression and ease anxiety.

Ginger: Ginger is a marvelous herb that promotes circulation, menstruation and also prevents delayed menstrual flow. In addition, ginger helps to settle the stomach and alleviate intestinal gas.

Ginseng: Of all the herbs, ginseng is most famous for its Oriental background and usage. It is excellent for treating and preventing fatigue and stress and works to alleviate depression. Ginseng is considered a glandular tonic.

Lady's Mantle: This herb helps to regulate the menstrual cycle with gentle hormonal action.

Milk Thistle: This helps regulate liver and kidney function.

Queen of the Meadow: This herb is a superb medicinal for its effective and gentle diuretic action. It also helps to alleviate kidney and bladder problems.

Sarsaparilla: This herb contains a natural source of progesterone.

Squaw Vine: Used for generations by Native American Women, Squaw Vine is good for its tryptophan content which is a precursor to serotonin. In order to combat the mood changes associated with PMS, adequate levels of serotonin must be produced within brain cells.

White Willow Bark: Considered a nerve sedative, this herb is used as a safe alternative to pharmaceutical pain killers and is used to treat uterine cramping and discomfort.

Wild Yam: This herb is very good for treating menstrual cramps.

ADDITIONAL HERBAL HELPS

Herbs for the Endocrine System: Burdock, Echinacea, Chaparral, Golden Seal, Red Clover, Licorice, Yellow Dock, Barberry, Dandelion, Peach, Oregon Grape, Yucca, Chickweed, and Watercress.

Herbs for the Circulatory System: Capsicum, Garlic, Hawthorne, and Rosemary.

Herbs for the Nervous System: Hops, Skullcap, Ho Shou-Wo, Wood Betony, Passion Flower, and Valerian Root.

Herbs for the Digestive System: Alfalfa, Kelp, Comfrey, Chamomile, Wild Yam, Papaya, Peppermint, Catnip, Spearmint and Fennel.

EXERCISE AND PMS

One very famous lady star recently stated on a popular talk show that if she had not embraced exercise during her struggle with menopause, she would have lost her mind. The beneficial effects of exercise on every body system are impressive to say the least. Exercise is a must for all women, but is especially good for those of us who suffer from hormonal upheavals and mood disorders. Exercise not only gets the circulation going, toxins moving and calories burning, it also stimulates the release of brain chemicals called endorphins, which just make us feel good about living.

Start with a plan that you know you can implement. Failure is out of the question so don't plan strenuous marathons at five in the morning. Just decide to walk briskly for 30 to 40 minutes, three to five days a week. If you can get outside then you also glean from the good effects of fresh air and sunshine, but if you can't then invest in a good treadmill. If a treadmill is not feasible for financial or other reasons, get a good exercise tape and put it in your VCR and go at it. Your local library probably carries a number of these tapes that you can check out (literally)! The point is that any who are physically able can and should be exercising as part of our everyday lifestyle. Until we do, we will battle the bulge and the blues. We were designed to move. Exercising facilitates the better function of all of our body systems. When we exercise, we eliminate better, we sleep better, we have more fatigue, less depression, more stamina, strength and we can even think clearer. It's not a big deal, so start . . . right now.

Case Study: Nancy's Story

The following is an interview I conducted with a friend who has suffered from severe PMS and other hormone-related complaints. It has only been recently that PMS has been scientifically recognized as a legitimate disorder. Its link to mental as well as physical impairment is now well documented. Deciding exactly how to treat this multi-faceted syndrome is difficult. Frequently, physicians disagree among themselves as to what constitutes the best treatment options. In reading Nancy's story, however, it becomes evident that a definite correlation exists between diet, exercise, nutrition and hormone-related disorders like PMS. Nancy is a 39-year-old mother of eight children.

LT: Nancy, how has your menstrual cycle affected your moods?
Nancy: I started my period early in the sixth grade. I don't remember feeling any different although my brothers used to always say, " Boy you sure can tell what day it is with Nancy.î I guess I became very grouchy during my periods and I also remember feeling sore when I ovulated. As I grew older, I began to have two periods a month and ovulation times became more obvious as far as mood changes go. I would become very sensitive, especially with those closes to me. After the birth of my twins, I went into a deep depression which lasted for two years. I was on anti-depressant drugs as well as progesterone therapy. I was also experiencing severe constipation.
LT: When did you first make the connection between your hormones and your mood swings?

Nancy: I always had physical side effects with my periods . . . headaches and bloating, but they became worse with the birth of each baby. I really began to connect my emotional symptoms with hormonal factors after my sixth baby, who was born when I was 32.

LT: How do you feel when you experience a hormone-related depression?

Nancy: Hormonal mood swings differ for me from a more typical kind of depression. During these periods of depression, I would actually begin to question the validity of my basic beliefs and values. Suddenly, the things that were the most important to me didn't seem to mean that much at all (church, family, friend, job, etc.). I also thought that anything that would make me feel better was okay.

LT: Have you experienced food cravings associated with your cycle?

Nancy: Yes, with ovulation, I craved salty foods and sweet things during my periods. The craving for chocolate and caffeine became almost insatiable.

LT: What kind of effect did the foods you ate have on how you felt?

Nancy: Caffeine products would give me an immediate emotional lift. By the time I was 30, I was so addicted to caffeine that I began to notice that it was really making things worse. It seemed to make my ovulation time much more painful. My doctors suspected that my ovulatory pain was caused by cysts that enlarge during the monthly cycle. I did have a major cyst and was hospitalized for six days due to complications caused by its presence. I realized then that I had to try to leave caffeine alone. When I eliminated caffeine from my diet, I found that I had no more ovulation pain. I also began to see a direct correlation with the use of sugar and PMS problems at this time. When I cut my sugar intake, problems with bloating and headaches disappeared. Chocolate has always been a problem for me. If I smelled chocolate on certain days of the month, it would give me a headache but I still craved it. One time I woke up at three o'clock in the morning and drove to a convenience store for a chocolate bar and a Pepsi. When I went on a diet with no sugar, fat or caffeine, I started my period without my typical headache or bloating for the first time.

LT: When was your PMS at its worse and why do you think it was?

Nancy: After the birth of my twins, I discovered that I was ovulating twice a month. This meant that my hormone activity was significantly higher than normal. In essence, my PMS problems doubled. I had been on high doses of caffeine in the form of soft drinks and pain killers during my pregnancies to help relive nausea and discomfort. My body had become depleted of B vitamins as well as other nerve-building nutrients. My PMS symptoms subsided the most when I eliminated sugar and caffeine from my diet and used vitamins and herbs.

LT: How did anti-depressant and progesterone therapy affect you?

Nancy: I gained ten pounds in nine days after I went on anti-depressants that stayed with me for over a year. I became less excited and ambitious on these drugs and my sexual drive diminished. I was also constantly tired. I took progesterone suppositories for six months. They were good in that I felt an immediate emotional improvement which let me know just how good I could feel. The side effects, however, were really severe and they were quite expensive. I found myself developing frequent yeast infections and in time, felt like the good effects of these drugs was wearing off.

LT: What effect did exercise have on your PMS symptoms?

Nancy: Exercise is wonderful. It helps regulate the emotions and cleans out the body at the same time. It's like blowing the carbon out of an old engine. In real cases of depression, however, your energy levels are so low that it is extremely hard to exercise. Personally, I found that exercise forestalled depression but was not a cure-all.

LT: What herbs and vitamins have your found to be helpful?

Nancy: Cascara Sagrada is a lower bowel cleansing herb which has really helped my constipation, which was a big part of my problem. Dong Quai helps me to relax and sleep better as well as contributing to more normal ovulation. It has also helped me regulate my periods. The B vitamins have helped my nerves. Yeast free B vitamins are the only ones I can tolerate. I also found the use of vitamins E, A, and D helpful. The herbs and vitamins are great supplements to a diet based on lots of fresh fruits and vegetables.

LT: Nancy, has it been worth all the effort and changes you have had to make?

Nancy: When you get to the point that your body is affecting your emotions so negatively that you feel everything you really care about is threatened, then it is definitely worth it. It's so hard to recognize that physical factors may be at the heart of your problems. Instead, you assume you're just becoming an unhappy, miserable person.

It's important to start with one thing and see if that makes a difference and then build from there. For example; avoid caffeine and take the appropriate vitamins and herbs. Feeling healthy is worth any effort for not only yourself, but those around you as well. My family means so much to me. It's such a good feeling to know that the good qualities I have can dominate the negative aspects of my personality. I can enjoy life and the people I love on a consistent basis.

COMMENTS ON NANCY'S INTERVIEW

Nancy's story may differ in some detail from the experience of other women, however, most of her experience is shared by those who cope with PMS. More and more doctors are beginning to look to diet, nutrition and exercise as crucial components in treating PMS. Depression ran in Nancy's family, therefore, brain chemistry may have compounded her problem. While alcohol may become of crutch for people prone to depression, Nancy found that sugar, caffeine, chocolate, red meats and fats were also addictive substances she felt she had to have to cope.

As a young girl, Nancy ate a good diet; however, after her teenage years, began to exist on fast foods and caffeine products. By the age of 17, Nancy was taking two to three pain relievers that contained caffeine every day. As a young mother, her diet improved, however the discomforts of pregnancy heightened her sugar and caffeine consumption. With the typical demands of a large family and several miscarriages, her body became depleted of the nutrients it needs to maintain physical and mental health. The very things she craved, were the foods and substances that hurt her the worst.

Equally important is the fact that Nancy had to accept that her problems were hormonally and nutritionally related before she could really begin to solve them. Nancy's husband was able to see the emotional effect of her cycles and even how she behaved 4 to 6 hours after consuming caffeine. He shares how Nancy would typically seem all right and them suddenly turn on him or begin to yell at the kids. It took sometime before he could trace her behavior back to the caffeine.

Nancy's husband saw what Nancy was really like on her good days. The contrast was so dramatic that he refused to accept the fact that the situation was hopeless. Once they both accepted that the problem existed, Nancy turned to drug therapy which only provided temporary relief and came with a variety of undesirable side effects. Fortunately, Nancy had the courage and the knowledge to change her diet and supplement her nutrition with vitamins, herbs and exercise. She began a little at a time and while there were the inevitable set backs of changing one's lifestyle, she persevered.

The rewards of Nancy's efforts were great. She discovered that she could control her moods and behavior. By making the necessary changes in her life, Nancy has been able to win the battle against PMS. She is back in control of her life and knows first hand how intrinsically linked the body and the mind are. All women need to evaluate how they feel and observe how their cycles affect their physical and mental health. Watch your entire cycle and look for patterns of depression, irritability, sore breasts etc. Experiment and find out what works for you. PMS is not just a fabricated excuse for negative behavior. It is a debilitating disease that can destroy the quality of one's life, family and future. Nancy chose to fight and she is winning.

Menus/Recipes for a PMS Prevention Diet

Remember, the PMS prevention diet emphasizes the use of *whole grains,* such as wheat, corn, barley, oats, rye, millet, buckwheat and brown rice; *legumes,* such as lentils, kidney beans, pinto beans, mung beans, garbanzo beans, adzuki beans, and split peas; *seeds and nuts,* such as raw or roasted sesame seeds, sunflower seeds, raw almonds, and pecans; *root vegetables* such as carrots and potatoes, and *leafy green vegetables* such as kale, collard and mustard greens (eat vegetables raw whenever possible); *fruits* in season (preferably eaten raw); *oils* such as sesame, olive and safflower; and *lean meats,* such as poultry and white fish.

DIET GUIDELINES

• Limit your consumption of refined foods made with white sugar and white flour, and other concentrated sugars found in syrups, dried fruits and sweet juices.
• Decrease your consumption of animal protein and get your protein from vegetable sources such as legumes.
• Greatly decrease your consumption of dairy products, especially milk.
• Limit your intake of fats and use only vegetable oils rich in linoleic acids.
• Greatly increase your intake of fresh, green, leafy vegetables.
• Use hormone free poultry.
• Use more fish instead of meat.
• Limit your salt intake
• Avoid caffeine, chocolate, alcohol and nicotine
• Greatly increase your intake of dietary fiber

The following are suggested menu plans and recipes taken from *Today's Healthy Eating,* by Louise Tenney. The recipes marked with an asterisk are included in this booklet.

Seven-Day Sample Menu

#1 Breakfast
*Buckwheat Crepes or pancakes with topping / Apple juice

#1   Lunch
*Broccoli Quiche / 10 raw almonds / vegetable juice

#1   Supper
*Layered Salad / *Sesame Bread Sticks

#2 Breakfast
*Super Breakfast Cereal w/ nut and seed milk / Red raspberry leaf tea

#2 Lunch
*Lentil soup / *Cheese cornbread

#2 Supper
*Winter vegetable salad / Whole grain bread

#3 Breakfast
Poached egg / Whole grain toast / Orange juice

#3 Lunch
*Stuffed Peppers / Vegetable Juice / Sunflower Seeds

#3 Supper
*Baked Rice and Miller / Steamed Carrot Slices

#4 Breakfast
*Mixed Fruit Compote / *Bran Muffin

#4 Lunch
*Bean Soup / *Millet Crackers / Carrot Slices

#4 Supper
*Vegetable Corn Chip Salad / Vegetable Juice

#5 Breakfast
*Raw Oat Cereal / 1/2 Grapefruit / Chamomile Tea

#5 Lunch
*Pineapple Waldorf Salad / 10 raw almonds

#5 Supper
*Minestrone Soup / *Cheese Corn Bread / Celery Sticks

#6 Breakfast
*Energy Drink / Blueberry Muffin

#6 Lunch
*Garden Salad with choice of dressing

#6 Supper
*Bean and Millet Supper / Steamed Broccoli

#7 Breakfast
*Raw Granola #2 / Apple/Chamomile Drink

#7 Lunch
*Spanish Millet Loaf / Steamed Broccoli

#7 Supper
*Vegetable Stir-Fry / Steamed Chicken Breast

Recipes

BREAKFAST

Buckwheat Crepes

1/2 C. buckwheat flour	1 C. milk
1/2 C. whole wheat pastry flour	1/2 C. water
1/4 C. wheat germ	1/2 tsp. mineral salt
3 eggs	3 T. cold-pressed oil

Combine flours, eggs, milk, water salt and oil. Mix in blender. Batter should be thick, but if it is too thick the crepe will curl up at the edges when cooking. Add more milk to batter if needed. Heat the skillet and spread butter and oil mixture on surface. Using butter alone will burn. Pour 1/3 cup of crepe batter onto pan and swirl to cover entire surface or tilt the pan to cover the bottom. Cook crepe about one minute and flip to cook other side. The second side does not need to be brown for it to be done.

Toppings Suggestions: Blueberry sauce with sour cream or whipping cream. Fresh strawberries are also good.

Super Breakfast Cereal

1/2 C. oatmeal	1/4 C. raw chopped almonds
1 C. plain yogurt	1 T. sesame seeds
2 T. orange juice	1/2 C. chopped peaches
1 T. honey	1/2 C. chopped apples
1/2 C. raisins	1/2 C. sliced bananas

Fold all ingredients together. You can substitute sunflower seeds for sesame seeds or pecans for almonds.

Mixed Fruit Compote

2 apples	thin slice of lemon
1 C. dried fruit	1/4 C. ground almonds
1/2 C. currants	1/2 lemon, juiced
1/2 stick cinnamon	

Slice apples in chinks and put in saucepan with all other ingredients except currants. Bring to a boil then simmer on low heat, covered, for about 30 minutes. Remove the cinnamon stick and lemon slice. Stir in currants and serve for breakfast. Makes 4 servings.

Raw Oat Cereal

1/2 C. baby oats	1 tsp. date sugar
1 T. ground almonds	1 T. raisins soaked in water
1 T. ground sesame seeds	

Add bananas, fresh peaches, fresh berries, ground sunflower seeds, sesame seeds, coconut and cashews. Add rice polishings, flaxseed meal, wheat germ and bran.

Energy Drink

8 oz. Papaya juice	1 T. wheat germ
1 fresh peach	1 T. chia seeds
2 T. protein supplement	2 oz. plain yogurt
1 T. rice polishings	1 T. sunflower seeds

Blend the above ingredients together. The papaya juice contains protein digestive enzymes. The addition of protein supplement provides protein and natural b-complex vitamins. The yogurt makes the drink more digestible and helps to prevent the formation of gas. The sunflower seeds offer nutrition and energy along with unsaturated fatty acids. The chia seeds also produce energy and are very high in vegetable protein.

Raw Granola #2

1 C. sprouted triticale	1 C. coarse ground almonds
1 C. ground sunflower seeds	10 T. apple juice
1 C. of ground sesame seeds	1 C. of chopped light figs
1 T. of chia seeds (soaked over night in apples juice)	1 C. dates

Mix all ingredients together and moisten with apple juice.

LUNCH

Broccoli Quiche

2 C. chopped broccoli
1 C. fresh sliced mushrooms
1/2 C. chopped onions
1 clove garlic, pressed
dash of nutmeg
1/4 C. minced parsley
dash of vegetable seasoning

1 C. half and half
1 1/2 C. grated Swiss cheese
1/2 tsp. mineral salt
1 tsp. basil
2 T. butter
6 beaten eggs

Saute broccoli, onions, and mushrooms in butter. Cook until onions are transparent. Mix eggs, cheese, salt, nutmeg, basil, parsley and vegetable seasoning. Pour into a buttered two quart casserole dish and bake for 30 minutes at 350 degrees F.

Lentil Soup

2 C. lentils
5 C. bran water
1 qt. Tomatoes
2 stalks celery, chopped
1 large green pepper

2 large carrots, chopped
2 cloves garlic, minced
1/2 tsp. basil
1/4 C. tamari
Kelp or vegetable seasoning to taste

Combine all ingredients except kelp in a slow cooker. Cover and cook on low heat for about 6 hours. Season to taste.

Stuffed Peppers

2 large green peppers, halved
1/2 C. chopped celery
1 C. water cress, chopped
1 tomato, chopped

3 green onions, chopped
1 C. peas, fresh or frozen
Homemade mayonnaise
2 hard cooked egg yolks

Let green peppers chill in cold water for a few hours. Mix all ingredients together and fill pepper halves just before you're ready to eat.

Bean Soup

1 C. navy beans
4 C. pure water
1 C. grated carrots
1 small onion, grated

1/2 C. chopped parsley
1 T. nut cream
1 tsp. lemon juice

Soak beans overnight in three cups of water. Cook bean in 4 cups of water until tender. Blend the cooked beans and vegetables in a blender. Add parsley, nut cream and lemon. Let boil for a few minutes and then serve.

Pineapple Waldorf Salad

1 C. celery hearts

1 C. apples

1 C. fresh pineapple

1/4 C. chopped walnuts

Raisins, optional

Homemade mayonnaise

Leaf lettuce

Combine celery hearts, apples, pineapple, nuts and raisins. Add mayonnaise. This salad is also delicious without mayonnaise. Place on leaf lettuce and serve.

Garden Salad

3 C. leaf lettuce, torn

1/2 C. fresh shelled peas

1/2 C. grated carrots

1/2 C. grated zucchini

ground almonds

1 C. mung bean sprouts

1 cucumber sliced

1/2 avocado

1/2 C. sunflower seeds and

Mix all ingredients together. Serve with herb dressing or dressing of your choice. You can top the salad with sliced, fresh mushrooms.

Spanish Millet Loaf

2 C. cooked millet

1 C. whole wheat bread crumbs

1 small can green chilies

1 C. canned tomatoes

2 beaten eggs

2 T. vegetable seasoning

2 T. olive oil

1 tsp. chili powder

Combine all ingredients together. Pour into a buttered loaf pan. Cook for 45 minutes at 350 degrees F. While cooking, baste with butter two or three times. Serve with salsa.

SUPPER

Layered Vegetable Salad

4 C. romaine lettuce leaves

1/2 C. ground sunflower seeds

1 C. buckwheat sprouts

1 C. buckwheat sprouts

1 small cucumber sliced

1 large tomato

1 small green pepper

1 avocado

1 C. alfalfa sprouts

This is a complete salad meal. It contains protein that is easily digestible along with plenty of vitamins, minerals and live enzymes. Use salad oil with fresh lemon juice for the dressing. Break up the lettuce and use half of it on the bottom of salad bowl. Layer half of the other ingredients, add the rest of the lettuce and then another layer of the same ingredients.

Sesame Bread Sticks (unleavened)

2 C. sifted whole wheat flour	3 T. cold-pressed oil
1 T. date sugar or honey	1/2 tsp. cinnamon
1/2 tsp. sea salt (optional)	3/4 C. cold water

Add all ingredients together and stir well. Knead and form into small balls. Roll into pencil-like strips 8" long and 1/2' around. Place on a greased cookie sheet. Sprinkle with sesame seeds and Bake for 30 minutes at 350 degrees F.

Winter Vegetable Salad

2 C. romaine lettuce	1 red pepper
2 C. leaf lettuce	1 green pepper
1 C. red cabbage	1 grated beet
1 C. cauliflower	1/4 C. green onions with tops
1 C. broccoli	1/2 C. ground sunflower seeds
1 C. grated carrots	

Dressing:

3/4 C. cold-pressed oil	1/2 tsp. paprika
1/4 C. fresh lemon juice	1 clove garlic, sliced
1/2 tsp. kelp	

Add all ingredients to a jar and shake well. Let sit for a few minutes so garlic can penetrate the oil. Garlic can be discarded before serving or it can be eaten.

Baked Rice and Millet

1 1/2 C. cooked brown rice	2 T. butter
1/2 C. cooked millet	1 T. tamari soy sauce
2 beaten eggs	1 C. chopped raw almonds
1 C. milk	1/4 C. chopped sunflower seeds

Mix all ingredients and pour into a 1 1/2 quart casserole dish. Bake for 30 minutes at 350 degrees F.

Vegetable Corn Chip Salad

3 C. torn lettuce
2 medium tomatoes diced
1/4 C. green onion
1 7 oz. can diced green chilies
1 1/4 C. cooked pinto beans

1 C. ripe avocado (optional)
1 C. fresh corn, cut off cob
1/2 C. diced ripe olives
2 C. unsalted, corn chips
1 C. grated mild cheese

Dressing:

° C. yogurt
° C. sour cream

4 T. French dressing
1 T. chili powder

Minestrone Soup

1 large can stewed tomatoes
1 Qt. Water
3 T. vegetable seasoning
1 large onion, chopped
2 C. sliced carrots
1/2 C. chopped celery
2 potatoes unskinned and diced
2 C. cooked pinto beans

1/2 C. uncooked millet
1 C. peas fresh or frozen
1/2 C. whole wheat pasta, broken up
2 T. minced, fresh parsley
2 bay leaves
1 tsp. mineral salt or kelp
2 T. cold-pressed oil (optional)
corn cut from one cob

Combine tomatoes, water, vegetable seasoning, onion, carrots, millet, parsley, bay leaves and mineral salt. Cook until millet is tender. Add rest of ingredients and cook for about 15 minutes more. Add oil before serving.

Cheese Corn Bread

2 eggs
1/4 C. cold-pressed oil
2T. minced onion
2 T. minced green pepper
2 tsp. baking powder

3/4 C. thick yogurt/sour cream
1/4 C. ground sesame seeds
1 C. yellow corn meal
2 C. grated cheddar cheese

Combine eggs and oil, blend well. Add other ingredients and mix. Grease an 8x8" pan and pour in batter. Bake at 350 degrees F. for about 40 minutes.

Bean and Millet Supper

1 C. cooked pinto beans
1 C. cooked milled
1/4 C. ground almonds
3 T. butter
1 C. chopped onions
1 C. chopped mushrooms

1/2 C. chopped celery
1 tsp. vegetable broth seasoning
3 tsp. lemon juice
dash of rosemary
dash of sage
1/2 C. green pepper

Saute the onions, peppers, mushrooms and celery in butter. Add seasonings and lemon juice with 1/2 C. of water. Cook on low heat for about 10 minutes. Add beans, millet and almonds. Makes 4 generous servings.

Vegetable Stir-Fry

1 C. sliced carrots	1/2 C. blanched/chopped almonds
1 C. red onions	1/4 C. sunflower seeds
1 C. sliced broccoli	2 T. Tamari soy sauce
1 C. cauliflower	1/2 tsp. basil
2 cloves minced garlic	1/4 tsp. cumin

Heat 2 tablespoons ghee, butter, or cold-pressed oil in wok or frying pan. Add carrots, onions, garlic, and herbs. Stir thoroughly; cover and let cook for 5 minutes. Stir occasionally; you may add a little of water if vegetables are too dry. Add broccoli and cauliflower, sunflower seeds and soy sauce and stir thoroughly, Cover and cook for about 2 minutes. Serve over millet, brown rice, or other grains. Use vegetables in season such as zucchini, green peppers, Brussels sprouts, or cabbage. Add fresh corn, mushrooms or bean sprouts.

Bran Muffins

1 C. bran	3/4 C. milk
1 1/2 C. whole wheat pastry flour	1/4 C. honey
1 ° tsp. baking powder aluminum free	2 T. cold-pressed oil
1 beaten egg	1 tsp. orange rind

Mix all ingredients together. Spoon batter into greased muffin tins. Bake for 20 minutes at 400 degrees F. or until muffins begin to pull away from pan. Makes a dozen muffins. For a special treat, grated fresh apples may be added to the batter.

Millet Crackers

1 T. dried yeast	1/2 C. dried light figs
1/2 C. lukewarm water	1 C. cold-pressed oil
1/2 C. hot water	3 C. millet flour
1/2 C. dried apricots	1 C. whole wheat pastry flour

Mix the yeast and lukewarm water. Pour the hot water in a blender and add apricots and figs, blending until the mixture is fine. Combine yeast and fruit together. Stir in the oil and the flours. Dough should be stiff. Add more flour if needed. Roll out to a thin layer on floured board. Cut into squares. Place on an oiled cookie sheet and let stand for 15 minutes before baking at 300 degrees F. for about 30 minutes.

Homemade Mayonnaise

1 C. safflower oil
2 egg yolks
2 T. fresh lemon juice
1 T. lecithin

1 1/2 T. apple cider vinegar
1 tsp. sesame kelp salt
1/4 tsp. mustard powder

Mix egg yolks in blender until thick. Add vinegar and blend for about 30 seconds. Pour the oil in while the blender is running very slowly, in a thin stream. Add lemon juice, sesame kelp salt, lecithin and dried mustard. Blend until smooth.

Bibliography

Downs,   Robert D.C.,   with Alice Van Back, "Natural Ways to Beat
    Premenstrual Tension,î Best Ways Magazine, December, 1983.

Elkins, Rita, Depression and Natural Medicine, Pleasant Grove, Utah:
    Woodland Publishing, 1995.

Laughlin, Mary, M.D. and Ramona E. Johnson, M.D., Premenstrual
    Syndrome, United Medical Centers, Santa Ana, California.

Murray, Michael, N.D. and Joseph Pizzorno, N.D., Encyclopedia of Natural
    Medicine, Rocklin, California: Prima Publishing, 1991.

Somer, Elizabeth, M.A., R.D. Nutrition for Women, New York: Henry Holt
    and Company, 1995.

Tenney, Louise, Today's Herbal Health, Pleasant Grove, Utah: Woodland
    Publishing.